Veterinary Medicine in Pakistan -2015

Haroon Rashid Chaudhry*, The Islamia University of Bahawalpur

Muhammad Javed*, UVAS, Lahore

Muhammad Asad, Khushi Muhammad, Masood Rabbani

Department of Microbiology, UVAS, Lahore-PAKISTAN

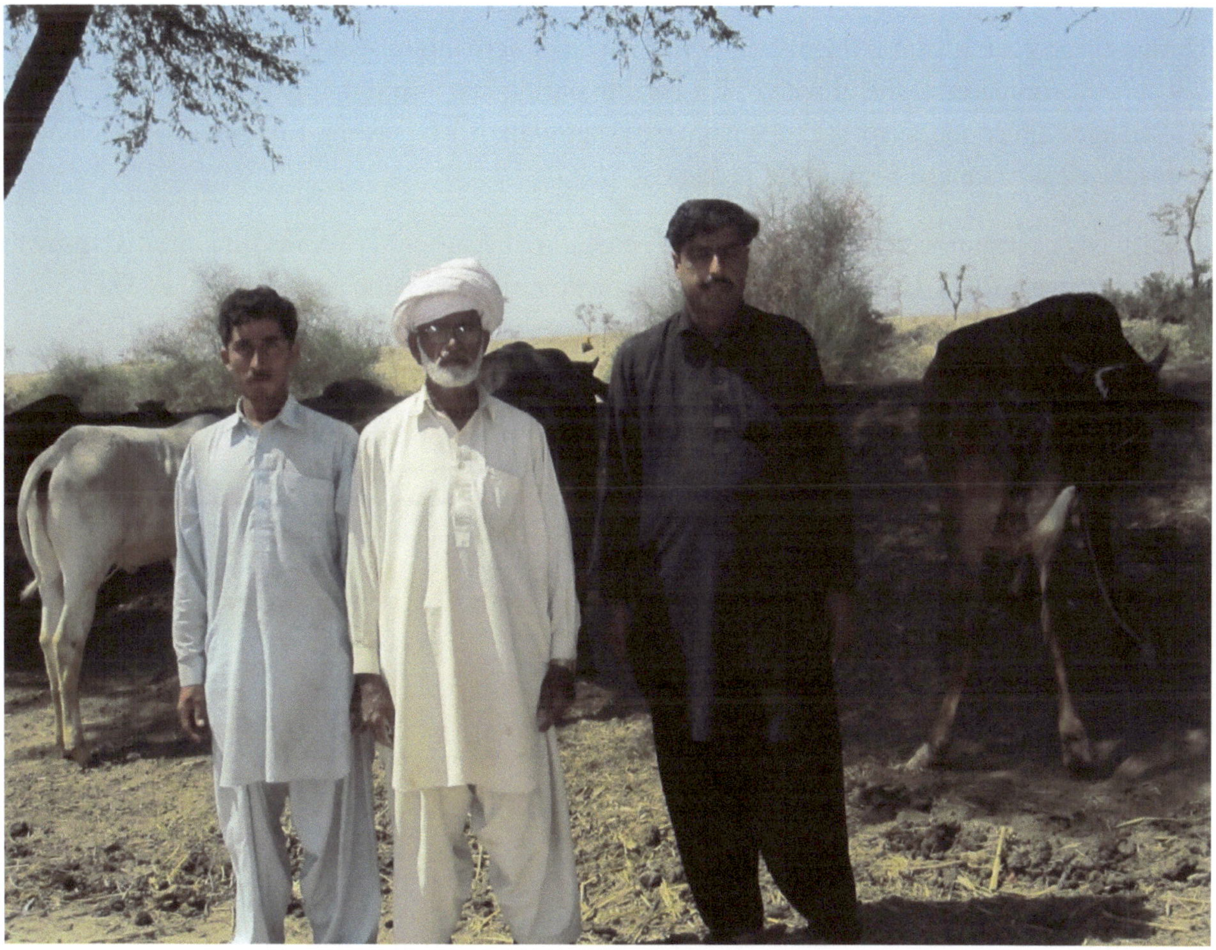

Agriculture and its role in Pakistan

Pakistan came into being in 1947. It has been a roller coaster ride since then. Pakistan originally designed as an agricultural state somehow went into being held by merchandisers and middlemen where no industrialist and no agriculturist is safe from their fate. This holds true even for the veterinary sector.

Agriculture accounted for 20.9 percent of the Gross Domestic Product (GDP) in 2014-15 and is a source of livelihood of 43.5 percent of rural population. Increased agricultural production and high crops yield is essential for food security which make the farming systems less vulnerable to climate change

During fiscal year 2014-15, the overall performance of agriculture sector recorded a growth of 2.9 percent compared to the growth of 2.7 percent during last year due to positive growth in all related agriculture sub sectors. Crops witnessed a growth of 1.0 percent, Livestock 4.1 percent, Forestry 3.2 percent and Fishing 5.8 percent.

The Livestock sector which contributes 56.3 percent in the agriculture recorded a positive growth of 4.1 percent in 2014-15 against 2.8 percent growth during the same period last year. The Fishing sector contributed 2.1 percent in agriculture value addition recorded a growth of 5.8 percent as against last year's growth of 1.0 percent. Forestry sector posted a growth of 3.2 percent this year as compared to the negative growth of 6.7 percent last year.

Table 2.1: Agriculture Growth Percentages (Base=2005-06)

Sector	2008-09	2009-10	2010-11	2011-12	2012-13	2013-14	2014-15 P
Agriculture	3.5	0.2	2.0	3.6	2.7	2.7	2.9
Crops	5.2	-4.2	1.0	3.2	1.5	3.2	1.0
i) Important Crops	8.4	-3.7	1.5	7.9	0.2	8.0	0.3
ii) Other Crops	0.5	-7.2	2.3	-7.5	5.6	-5.4	1.1
iii) Cotton Ginning	1.3	7.3	-8.5	13.8	-2.9	-1.3	7.4
Livestock	2.2	3.8	3.4	4.0	3.5	2.8	4.1
Forestry	2.6	-0.1	4.8	1.8	6.6	-6.7	3.2
Fishing	2.6	1.4	-15.2	3.8	0.7	1.0	5.8

Source: Pakistan Bureau of Statistics
P: Provisional

Veterinary Industry and its role in Pakistan

Livestock is an important sector of agriculture and occupies a unique position in the National Agenda of the economic development of the present government. The sector meets the domestic demand of milk, meat and eggs. It also provides net source of foreign earnings. More than 8.0 million rural families are involved in raising livestock. It is central to the livelihood of the rural poor in the country and can play an important role in poverty alleviation and can uplift the socioeconomic conditions of our rural masses.
Livestock contributed to agriculture value added stood at 56.3 percent while it contributes 11.8 percent to the national GDP during 2014-15 compared to 55.6 percent and 11.8 percent during

the same period last year, respectively. Gross value addition of livestock has increased from Rs. 778.3 billion (2013-14) to Rs. 801.3 billion (2014-15), recorded an increase of 3.0 percent as compared to previous year. The livestock population for the last three years is given in Table 2.21.

Table 2.21: Livestock Population			(Million Nos.)
Species	2012-13[1]	2013-14[1]	2014-15[1]
Cattle	38.3	39.7	41.2
Buffalo	33.7	34.6	35.6
Sheep	28.8	29.1	29.4
Goat	64.9	66.6	68.4
Camels	1.0	1.0	1.0
Horses	0.4	0.4	0.4
Asses	4.9	4.9	5.0
Mules	0.2	0.2	0.2

Source: Ministry of National Food Security & Research
1: Estimated Figure based on inter census growth rate of Livestock Census 1996 & 2006

The major products of livestock are milk and meat which for the last three years are given in Table 2.22.

Table:2.22 Milk and Meat Production			(000 Tonnes)
Species	2012-13[1]	2013-14[1]	2014-15[1]
Milk (Gross Production)	**49,400**	**50,990**	**52,632**
Cow	17.372	18.027	18.706
Buffalo	30.350	31.252	32.180
Sheep[2]	37	38	38
Goat	801	822	845
Camel[2]	840	851	862
Milk (Human Consumption)[3]	**39,855**	**41,133**	**42,454**
Cow	13.897	14.421	14.965
Buffalo	24.280	25.001	25.744
Sheep	37	38	38
Goat	801	822	845
Camel	840	851	862

Table:2.22 Milk and Meat Production			(000 Tonnes)
Species	2012-13[1]	2013-14[1]	2014-15[1]
Meat[4]	**3,379**	**3,531**	**3,696**
Beef	1.829	1.887	1.951
Mutton	643	657	671
Poultry meat	907	987	1074

Source: Ministry of National Food Security & Research

1: The figures for milk and meat production for the indicated years are calculated by applying milk production parameters to the projected population of respective years based on the inter census growth rate of Livestock Census 1996 & 2006.

2: The figures for the milk production for the indicated years are calculated after adding the production of milk from camel and sheep to the figures reported in the Livestock Census 2006.

3: Milk for human consumption is derived by subtracting 20% (15% wastage in transportation and 5% in calving) of the gross milk production of cows and buffalo.

4: The figures for meat production are of red meat and do not include the edible offal's.

The production of other livestock products for the last three years is given in Table 2.23.

Table: 2.23 Estimated Livestock Products Production

Species	Units	2012-13[1]	2013-14[1]	2014-15[1]
Eggs	Million Nos.	13.813	14.556	15,346
Hides	**000 Nos.**	**14,410**	**14,868**	**15368**
Cattle	000 Nos.	7.258	7.532	7,816
Buffalo	000 Nos.	7,050	7,232	7,447
Camels	000 Nos.	102	104	105
Skins	**000 Nos.**	**50,713**	**51,872**	**53,060**
Sheep Skin	000 Nos.	10,873	11,001	11,132
Goat Skin	000 Nos.	24,986	25,664	26,359
Fancy Skin	000 Nos.	14,854	15,207	15,569
Lamb skin	000 Nos.	3,229	3,268	3,306
Kid skin	000 Nos.	11,624	11,939	12,263
Wool	000 Tonnes	43.6	44.1	44.6
Hair	000 Tonnes	24.4	25.1	25.8
Edible Offal's	000 Tonnes	363	373	383
Blood	000 Tonnes	61.3	62.8	64.4
Guts	000 Nos.	51,232	52,403	53,603
Casings	000 Nos.	15,333	15,817	16,347
Horns & Hooves	000 Tonnes	52.5	54.0	55.5
Bones	000 Tonnes	780.5	802.9	827.2
Fats	000 Tonnes	248.8	255.8	263.3
Dung	000 Tonnes	1,104	1,136	1,171
Urine	000 Tonnes	338	348	358
Head & Trotters	000 Tonnes	226.3	232.3	238.8
Ducks, Drakes & Ducklings	Million Nos.	0.5	0.5	0.5

Source: Ministry of National Food Security & Research

1: The figures for livestock product for the indicated years were calculated by applying production parameters to the projected population of respective years.

Poultry Industry and its role in Pakistan

Poultry sector is one of the organized and vibrant segments of agriculture industry of Pakistan. This sector generates employment (direct/indirect) and income for about 1.5 million people. Poultry meat contributes 28.0 percent of the total meat production in the country. The current investment in Poultry Industry is more than Rs. 200.00 billion. Poultry sector has shown a robust growth @ 8-10 percent annually which reflects its inherent potential. This sector has contributed 1.3 percent in GDP during 2014-15 while it's contribution in agriculture and livestock value added stood at 6.3 percent and 11.2 percent, respectively. The poultry value added at current factor cost has increased from Rs. 130.7 billion (2013-14) to 140.5 billion (2014-15) showing an increase of 7.5 percent as compared to previous year. The production of commercial and rural poultry and poultry products for the last three years is given in Table 2.24.

Table 2.24: Domestic/Rural & Commercial Poultry				
Type	Units	2012-13[1]	2013-14[1]	2014-15[1]
Domestic Poultry	**Million Nos.**	**80.87**	**82.08**	**83.32**
Cocks	Million Nos.	10.38	10.66	10.95
Hens	Million Nos.	38.78	39.47	40.18
Chicken	Million Nos.	31.72	31.95	32.19
Eggs[2]	Million Nos.	3.878	3.947	4.018
Meat	000 Tonnes	108.62	110.79	112.99
Duck, Drake & Duckling	**Million Nos.**	**0.52**	**0.50**	**0.48**
Eggs[2]	Million Nos.	23.13	22.17	21.25
Meat	000 Tonnes	0.70	0.67	0.65
Commercial Poultry	**000 Tonnes**	**47.0**	**50.1**	**53.4**
Layers	Million Nos.	37.25	39.86	42.65
Broilers	Million Nos.	656.72	722.39	794.63
Breeding Stock	Million Nos.	9.71	10.19	10.70
Day Old Chicks	Million Nos.	685.94	754.54	829.99
Eggs[2]	Million No's	9.912	10.586	11.307
Meat	000 Tonnes	797.47	875.24	960.65
Total Poultry				
Day Old Chicks	Million Nos.	718	786	862
Poultry Birds	Million Nos.	785	855	932
Eggs	Million Nos.	13.813	14.556	15.346
Poultry Meat	000 Tonnes	907	987	1074

Source: Ministry of National Food Security & Research

1 : The figures for the indicated year is statistically calculated using the figures of 2005-06.

2 : The figures for Eggs (Desi) and Eggs (Farming) is calculated using the poultry parameters for egg production.

Losses incurred during 2014 in Livestock Industry

The flood hit the country in 2014. Punjab was the most affected area. Punjab Government took immediate measures to mitigate the losses in livestock sector. It established 642 emergency relief camps and 86 mobile dispensaries in the flood hit areas. The emergency vaccinations were done to 13.5 million large / small ruminants and 5.5 million rural poultry. Prophylactic treatment was provided to 14.5 million livestock. Since flood destroyed crops in many of the areas thus more than one lac Kgs Vanda was distributed in the flood affected areas to meet day to day need of livestock feeding. The economical losses to livestock sector were estimated to be more than Rs. 350 million.

Major holding situation of Livestock Industry

The Livestock Industry of Pakistan is at large a business of the poor. In this industry you will find a blind old woman with her grandchildren solely dependant on the three goats and male kid for their milk and six backyard poultry for the eggs. In this industry you will also be able to meet a small animal holding of 10-20 animals for milk and meat. These animals are fed on fodder from the small land holding they possess. Sheep and goat hererds are at large all throughout the country these shephards have a holding of 10-50 animals which feed on the roadside grasses and garbage from human waste. In villages they feed on the grasses and shrubs grown on the paved or unpaved roads and kacha besides the land divisions and no fodder is grown for them.

Metronamds are at large in small cities which feed on garbage sites of human waste. Goats take a liking for the small trees and shrubs grown besides the roads. Camels are reared in large number in deserts of cholistan and thar where camel holding ranges from 10-100s and they are all dependant on the thorny bushes and rare trees grown in the desert no proper feeding pattern is observed and these nomads change positions and possess little land holding. Besides the river tracts the nomads have a cattle holding of higher number ranging from 100-500s and they all are dependant on the riverine forest or the bushes that grow there their tract is well defined and usually reared by small children the animals are well familiar with their feeding and watering tract and in the evening they return to their base farm with little or no assistance these places are called bailas and kacha. Major population holding is in this area which when flood hit can cause major damage to the livestock. These bailas and kacha are well known for robberies and a best place for robbers and lootters which can steal the animals from villages and add to their number mostly stolen animals are found in this area. No branding and tagging is observed in Pakistan.

With the advent of commercialization by Nestle, Engro foods, Haleeb and rest of the others their has been a focus of industrialization of this industry. Although this is fake and yet very immature. They are being nurtured by high price of packed and processed milk and milk products as compared to the local gwallas. Not much work has been done on the viability of this industry but the writer thinks that this industry is standing on fake grounds where the profit is being managed by the gwallas and milk providers by adulteration of milk by water and the bigger agencies by the hike in price of the milk and milk products. This may be due to the lack of fodder and feed area where cheaper fodder can be grown for the animals. The milk is also adulterated by goat milk and sheep milk in which the only taxing cost is the migration of these animals along roadside and actually no cost comes to feeding. The writer may be unaware or the economics of the livestock is not yet balanced whatever the reason may be but it is a beneficial business because if the farm is leased from a bank and the owner has other sources of income and industry it serves as the best source of income to cut on taxation and leasing.

Cows, Buffaloes and Camels and their role in Pakistan
Milk is sold at a price of 60 rupees per liter in the rural and pre-urban area of Pakistan like Yazman and at a price of 60-70 rupees per liter in urban area like Lahore. While Packed milk is sold at Rs. 120 per liter.
A long list of factors account for this.
Unplanned breeding & Use of inferior bulls for breeding,
Lactation yields of dairy animals are significantly lower than many established breeds of exotic dairy cattle. There have been no consistent, systematic long-term programs aimed at improving genetic potential of local dairy animals. There is an extreme shortage of progeny tested bulls with high potential of milk cannot be purchased from known sources. Use of inferior bull for

mating in a very artless manner is the routine practice among the local farmers.

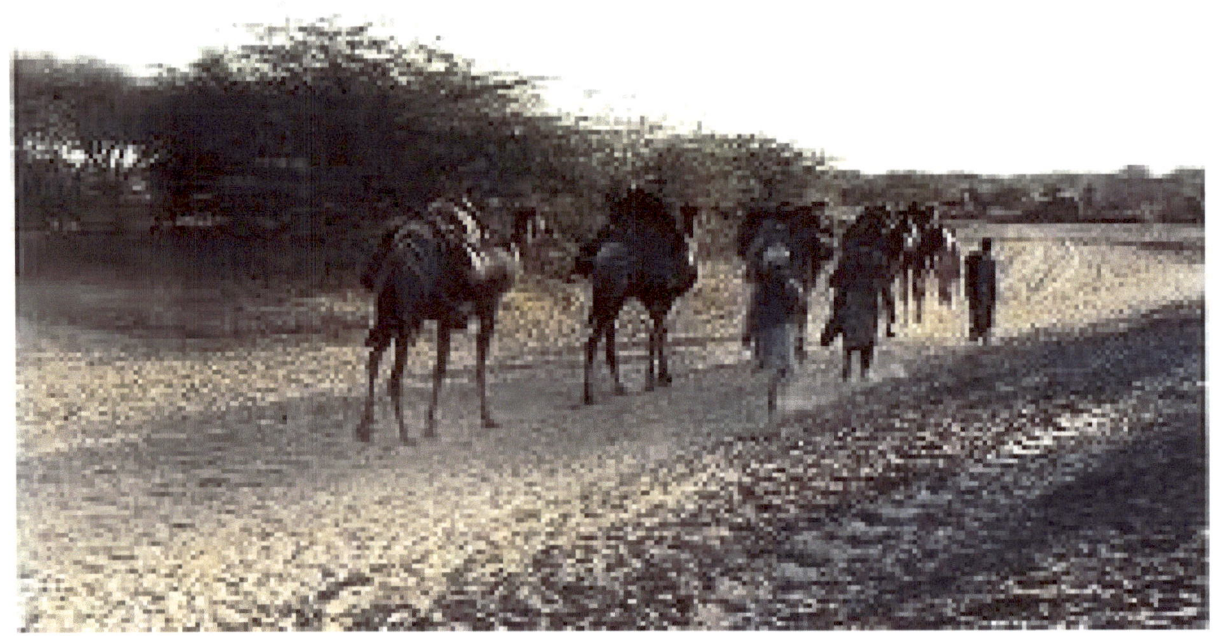

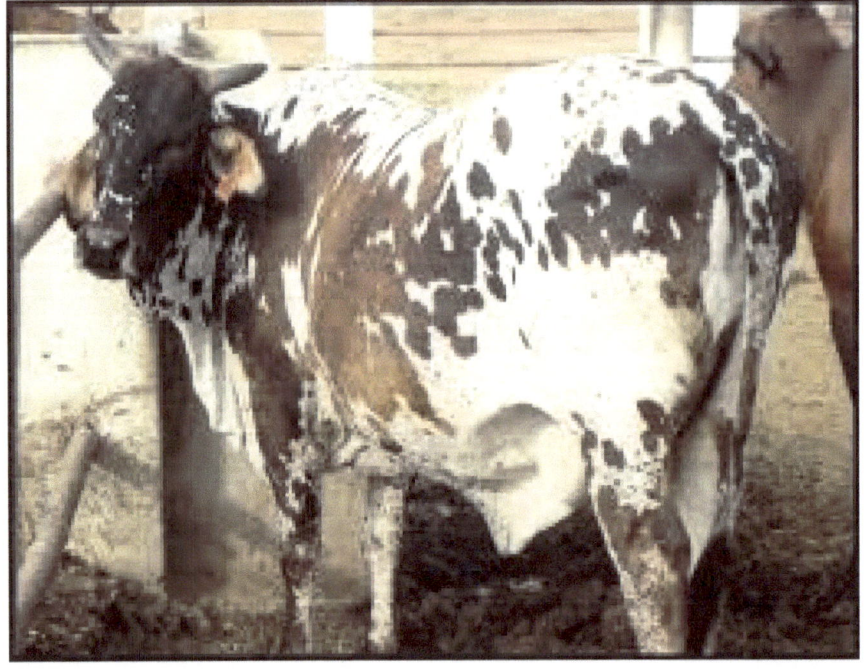

Informal production

In the age of modern science and technology while the world is using latest techniques in the livestock farming, the Pakistani farmer is still committed to their old practices in farming resulting in lower production per animal.

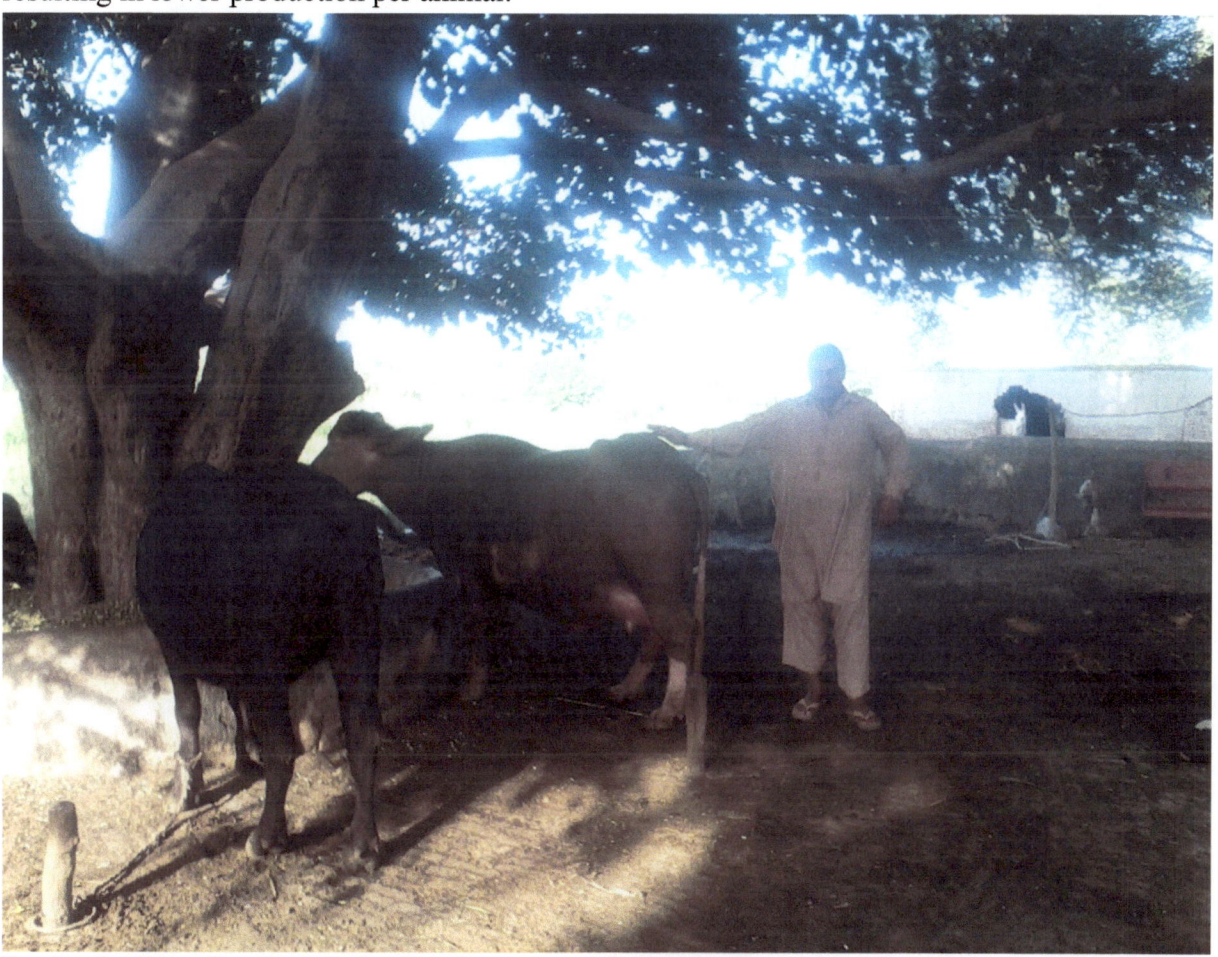

Lack of milk collection chain, involvement of middle man,

Proper marketing system encourages the animal productivity. Poor marketing system is also a significant constraint in the animal productivity. Private sector has organized the farmers' association for their own interest. These associations collect milk for the organizations. Regarding marketing farmers are on the mercy of beoparies and dodhies. These market players exploit the poor farmers. There should be systematic marketing system which could ensure the profit share of the farmers.

Inadequate feed resources and Seasonality,

An inadequate feed resource is the major constraint in the livestock sector for example, Cholistan, a large barren desert is dependent upon rain for its water supply and in turn its feed resources. This seasonal availability of water makes this area a seasonal pasture. Seasonal feed supply results in discontinues milk production which is not favorable for profitable enterprise.

Epidemics of infectious diseases,

No significant progress in reducing the overall mortality of livestock due to infectious diseases has made in this area. Foot and Mouth disease, Hemorrhagic Septicemia, black quarter and mastitis are still rampant in the Pakistan. These diseases not only cause heavy losses in terms of morbidity and mortality but also restrict export of livestock and livestock products.

Low investment and less interest of authorities,

Most of the governments have failed to realize the potential of Pakistan for livestock production. Public sector investments in the livestock sector have been pathetically low. Most of the governments have invested in short term projects and long term programs like genetic improvement of local cattle and buffaloes have generally been neglected.

Limited credit availability

Credit availability to the livestock sector has always been a problem. Most of the credit requirements are met from informal sector. As most of the livestock owners are small and landless farmers, collateral has been a major issue for them to have access to formal sector. Absence of a regular scheme of livestock insurance also shies the banks away

High temperature,

The climate of the area is an arid subtropical with low and sporadic rainfall, high temperature, low relative humidity. It is one of the driest and hottest areas of Pakistan, situated at 112m above the sea level with the mean annual temperature of 28.33°C. The month of June is the hottest when the daily maximum temperature normally exceeds 45°C, sometimes crossing 50°C.

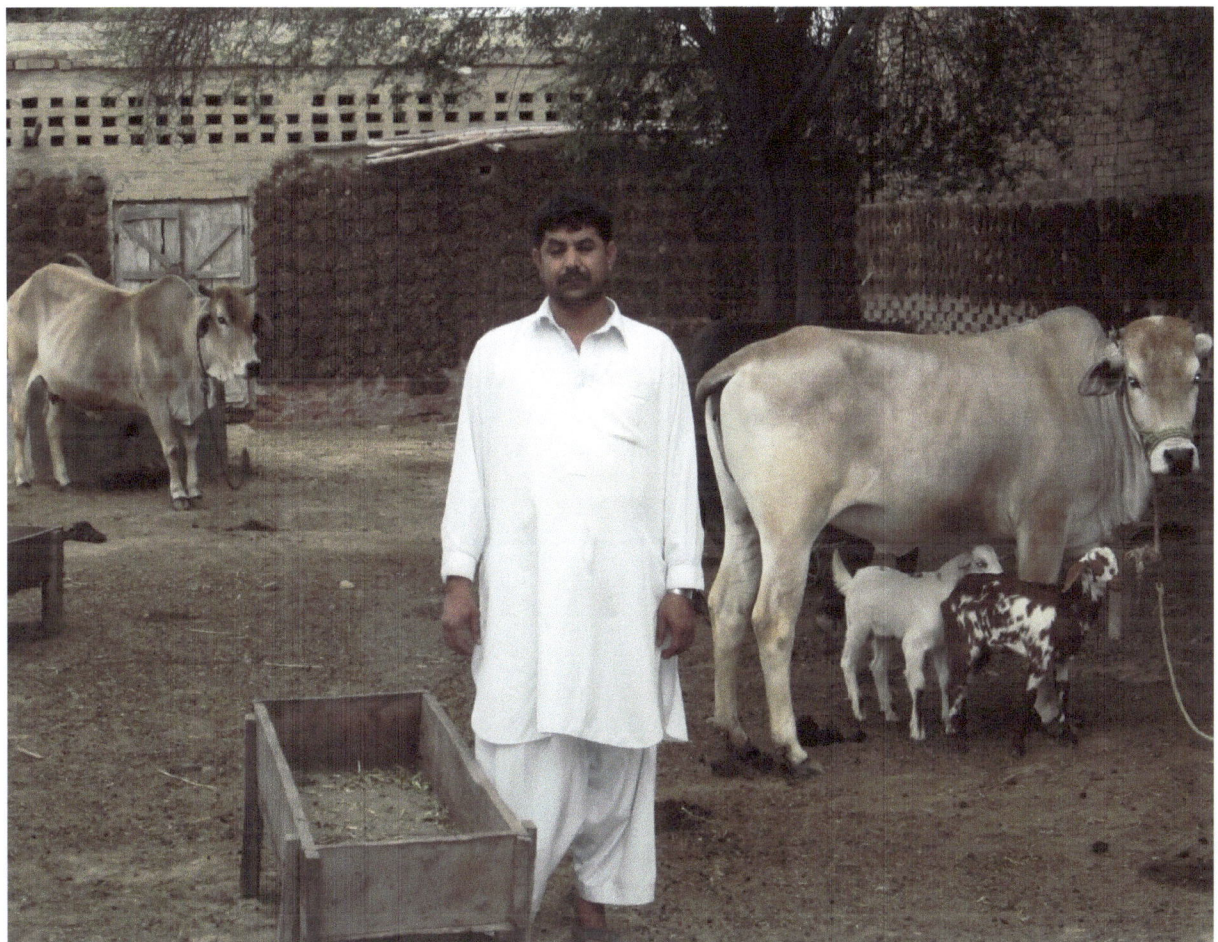

Many other factors which fall in constraints of dairy industry of Pakistan are:

- Lack of co-operation between local farmers.
- Lack of infrastructure
- Improper methods for preservation of milk,
- Unavailability of market,

Conclusion.

These problems can only be solved by long term planning by the government focusing on improvement of dairy sector by providing technical and financial assistance to the local farmers and developing interest of large stack holders for investing in this area.

Shepp and Goats and Metronomads

Families and Numbers

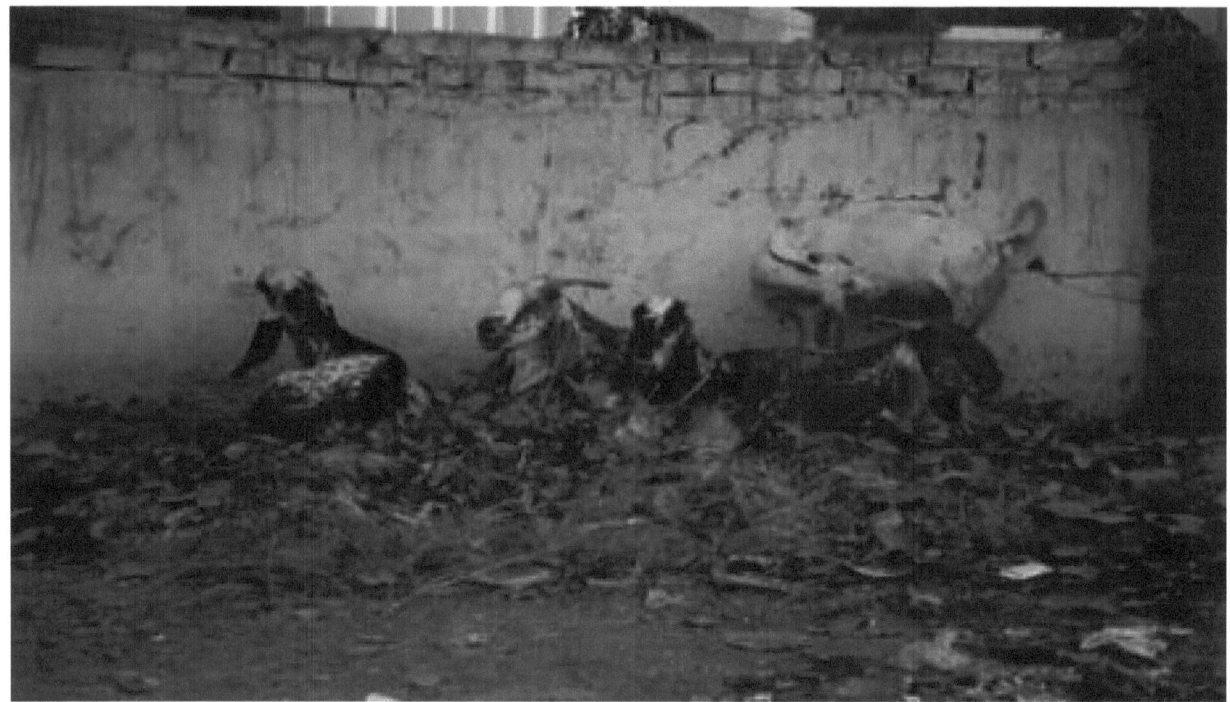

There are about 200 such families operating in the developing/developed suburbs of the cities. Hosting 25 and100 sheep and Goats of mixed variety respectively. The families live in a joint family system housing the elder parents and 5-6 mature married siblings with their children.

Age and Sex of Shepherds

These shepherds come in all ages and sizes but mostly are the young boys and girls. Female

Most of the flocks with these shepherds are unique in the sense that they comprised of sheep, goat and cattle. Sheep flock was comprised of 40% of the total participation is a must and 75% of the shepherds are females, even the mentally retarded female or male teenager will actively participate in this daily run to fetch food for the household.

herd

(mostly Khadri/Buchi breeds). While goat contributed 40-45% of the total herd (Mostly Beetle,

Cheeni, Nachi, Teddy random crosses). Almost 5% was constituted mixed Cholistani cattle or a Cholistani/Sahiwal cross.

Travelling and Time of Shepherding

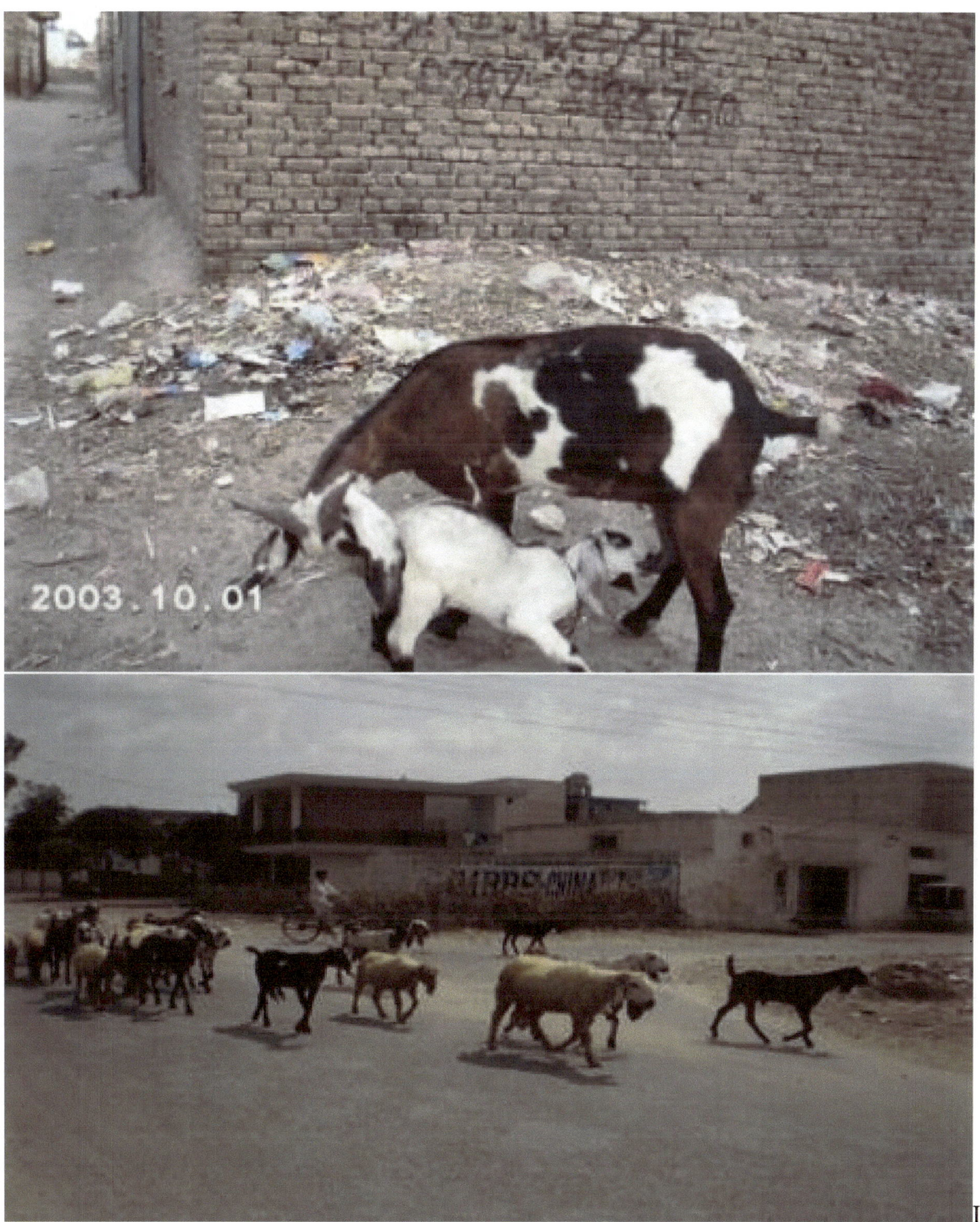

nteresting fact about the Pakistani system of nomading is that the goats are shepherded on the roads and they have located specific tracts for each shepherd's goats. The day starts at 4.00 am and the sheep and goats graze the garbage sites located in the 5-10 km radius. The evening round starts at 4.00 pm till the goats are furnished with food through the day.

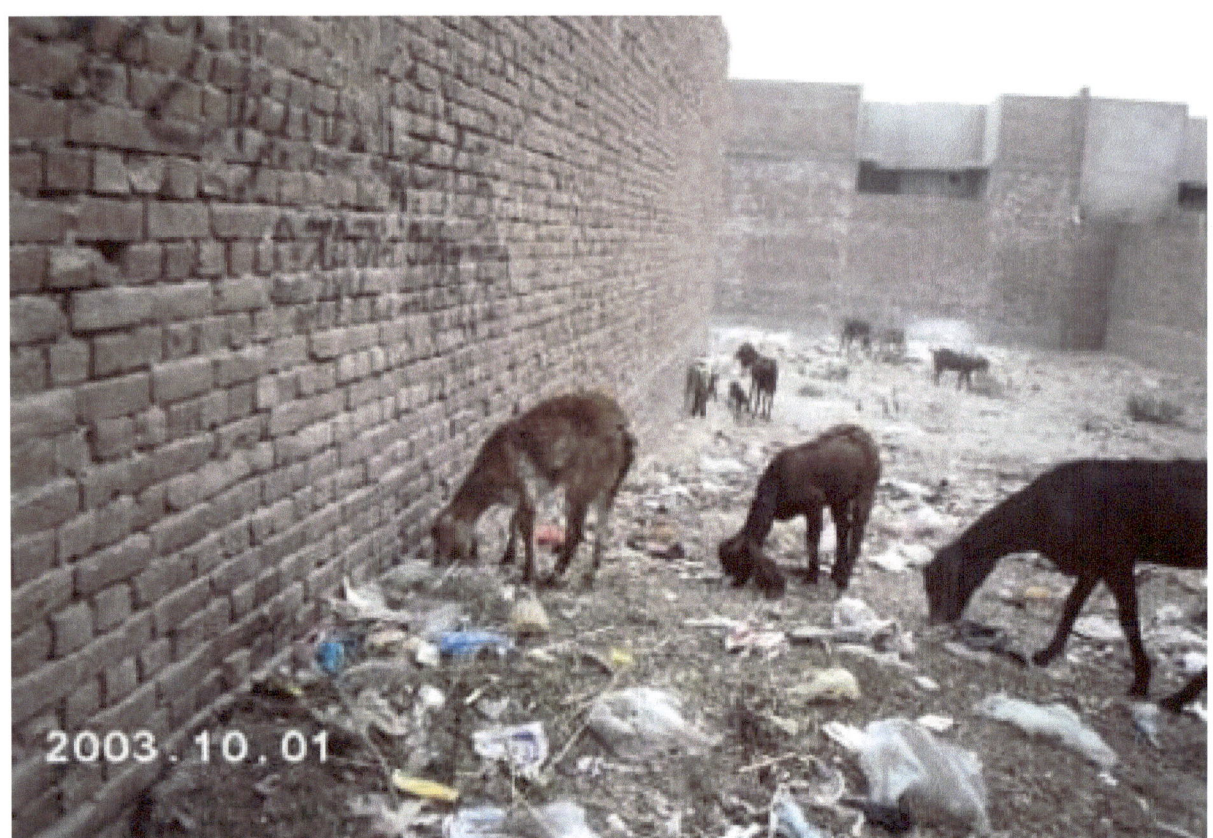

2003.10.01

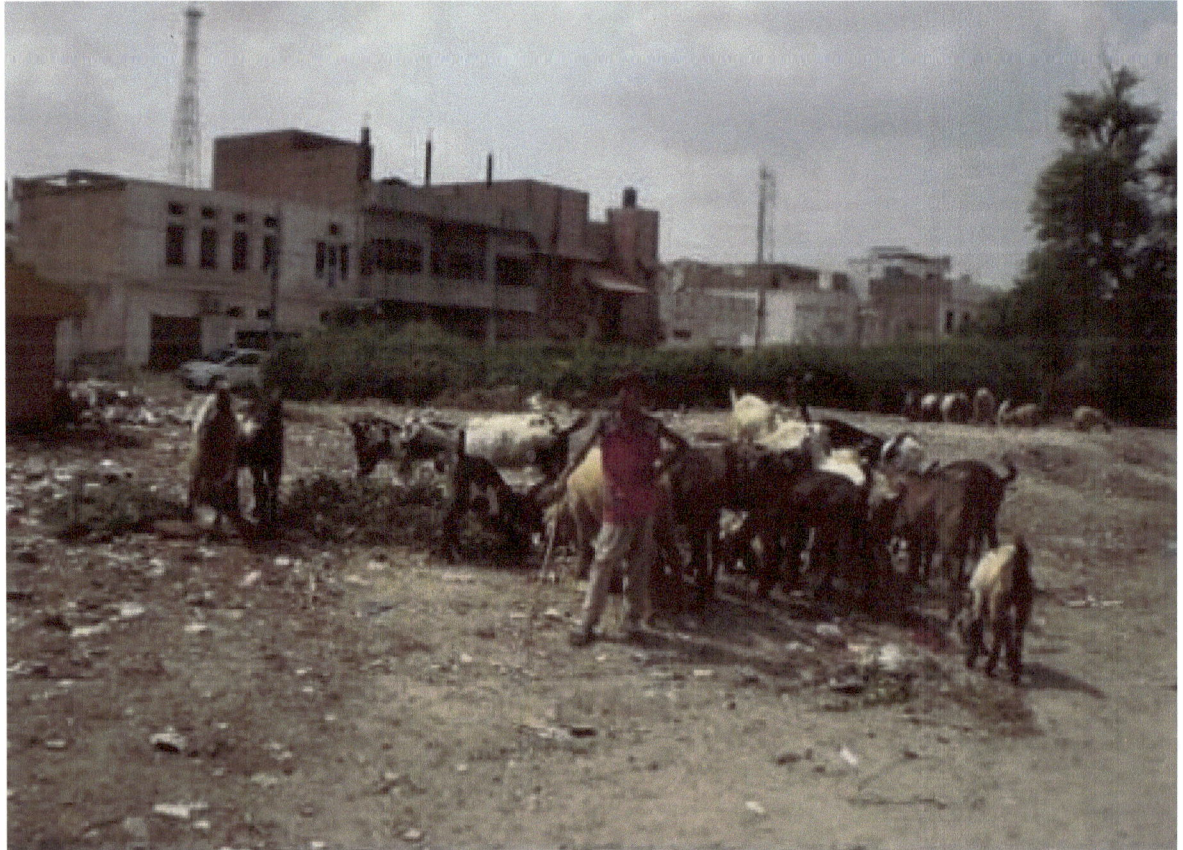

Most of the sheep and goats in a herd were mature and of breeding age with the exact

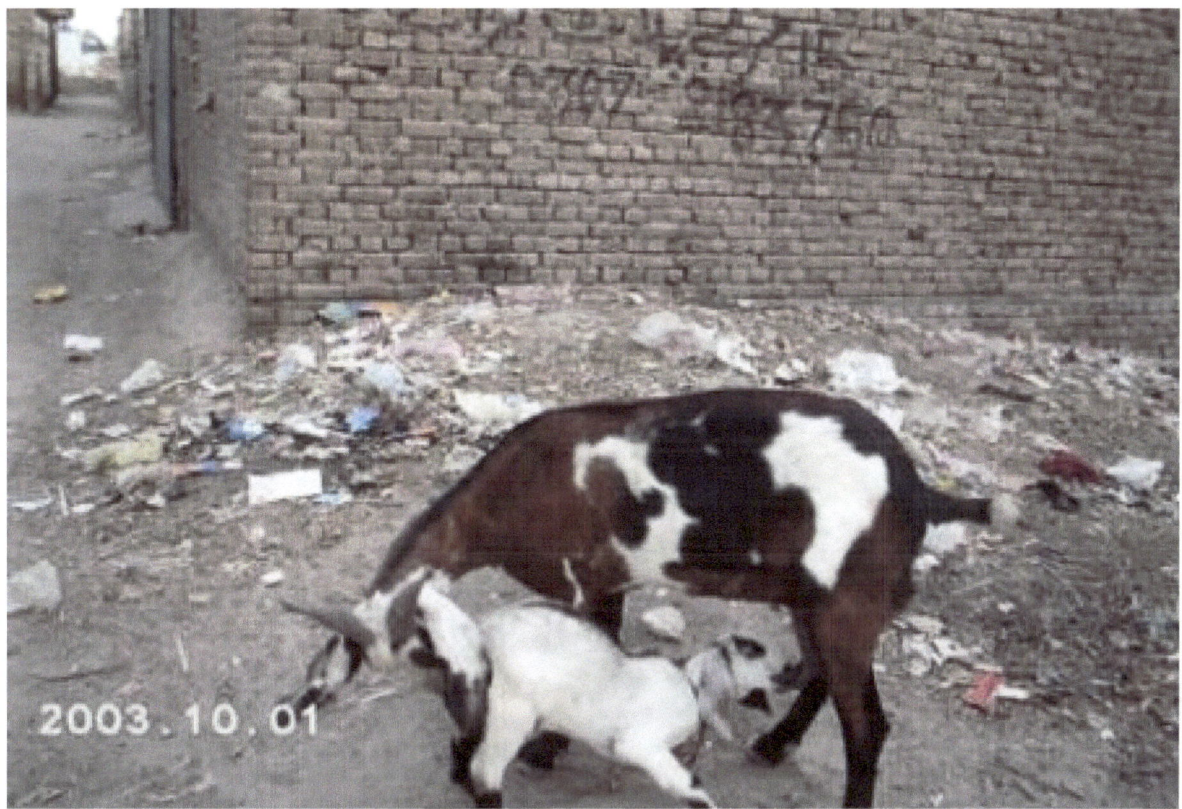

number of young ones which are reared in the house till weaning and are mature enough to traverse the city roads. 3-4 male sheep and goats are also part of the herd and they usually look after the herd and serve the female goat during oestrus.

Nutrition

The goats and sheep graze the municipal garbage disposal tankers where the garbage is posted along theside of the tankers and not in it. The sheep and goats eat the human waste like cut vegetable peelings, tea leftover, leftover food items, fruit peelings, dried fallen leaves and even disposed off papers, baby pampers. A day without such feasting is alternated by cutting down a branch of green tree by a shepherd blade/pole. The daily cost of food for the animals is Rs. 0/- for that day and minimal feed cost results in good profit.

Benefit Cost Ratio

Due to low or none feeding cost, after sale of milk and pathas an average monthly income of Rs. 40,000/- is minimum as far as 35 healthy productive goats are concerned.

Females supply around 1 to 2 litres of milk in a day. This milk is sold at the local tea stalls and milk stalls which are mixed with the cow/buffaloe milk and blended together after boiling. A herd normally of 25 female goats produce about 25-50 litres of milk which is sold in the market @ Rs. 15-20/liter (2010) and Rs. 25-30.00/liter (2011) bringing in daily bread and butter on regular basis. Larger herd means more money.

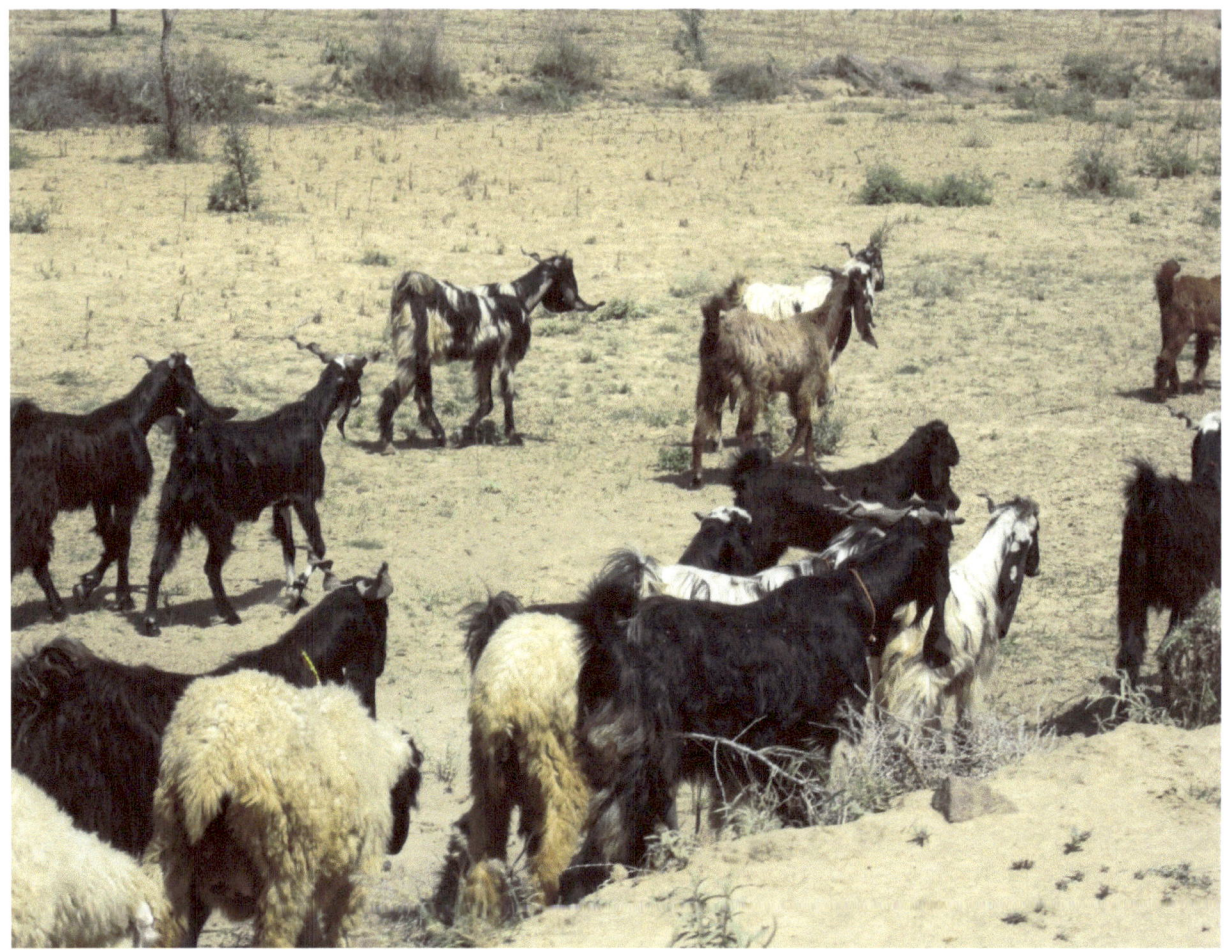

Male kids called pathas are sold at age of 6 months (Rs. 3,000/kid) to 1 year (Rs. 8-10,000/kid) to the local butchers. Older pathas are sold at age of 1-2 years to the local butcher @ Rs. 8-10,000/patha this need is felt for household emergency or in the case of sick animals.

Poultry

Poultry sector is one of the most organized and vibrant segments of agriculture industry of Pakistan. This sector generates direct and indirect employment and income for about 1.5 million people. Its contribution in agriculture and livestock is 6.4 percent and 11.5 percent, respectively. Poultry meat contributes 25.8 percent of total meat production in the country. Current investment in the poultry industry is about Rs 200.00 billion. The sector is showing a robust growth of 8 to 10 percent annually, which reflects its inherent potential. Poultry industry in its current year (2012) has produced 13114.00 million commercial eggs and 834,000.00 tons of poultry meat.

Poultry has emerged as a leading industry because it was developed by poorest for the poor which ranged in farm strength starting from 1,000 birds to 10,000 flock size at a farm site. Since the last decade especially post bird flu era the major industrialists have shown interest in poultry farming as a lucrative business and have invested in the construction of control sheds with size ranging from 30,000 birds to 120,000 flock size at a farm. With the advent of modern intensive

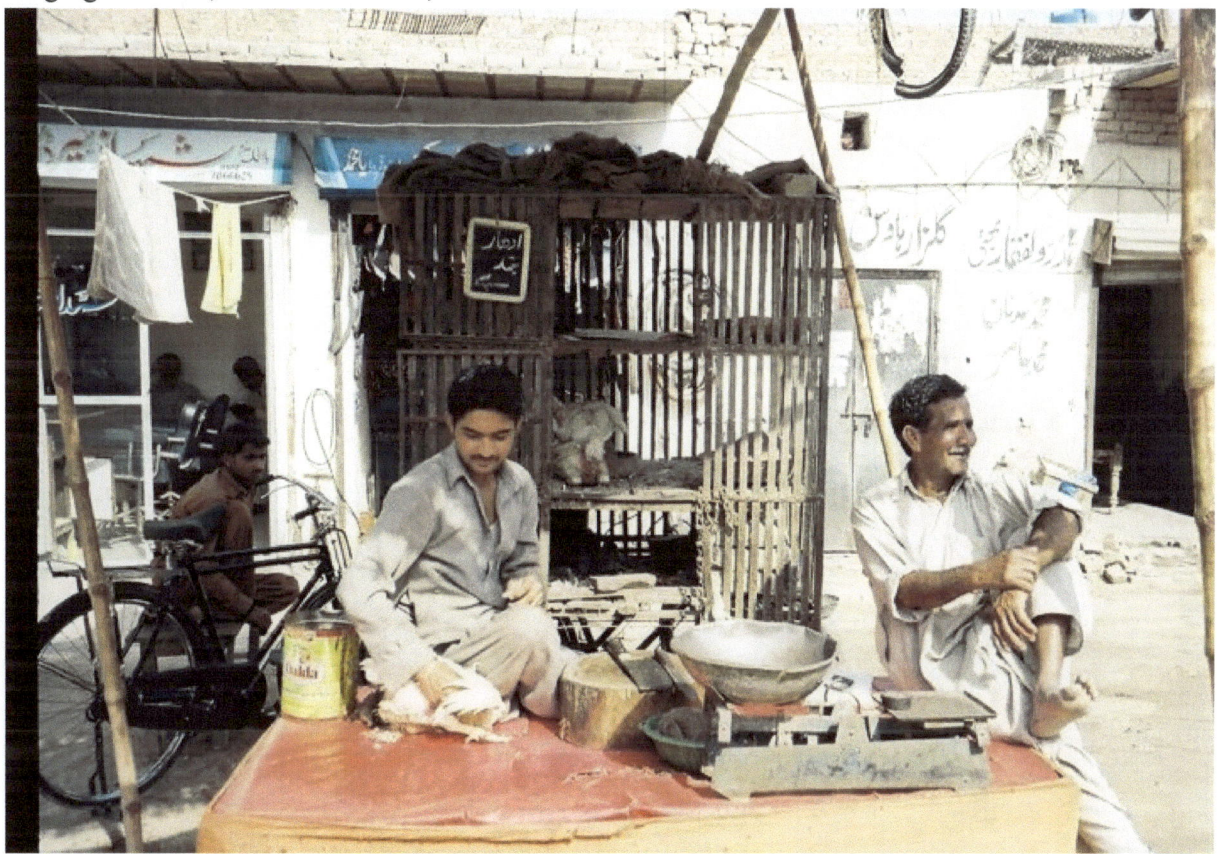

farming techniques in Pakistan, new challenges in disease protection and disease cure have emerged and posted a daunting challenge to the veterinarians and farm managers alike. Modern day practices in poultry farming have emerged without any laws governing their building design, place, farm to farm distance and have led to mushrooming effect sprouting in certain localities closer to major metropolitan cities.

Poultry industry has led to activities of slaughter phata's which is a unique feature in itself to the region of sub-continent. To picture a poultry slaughter unit I have posted some pictures of the slaughtering techniques used in Pakistan.

Ownership

Slaughtering phatas are usually owned by laymen and they pose a threat to the human health. Complete lack of resources in terms of money they start their business and the need to attain slaughtering technique or education is not required. Usually the laymen use boys who start to train as slaughtermen and when they mature they sit on the money box with a new face for cutting and slicing. To what extent is the food Halal is another question to be asked by molvi's.

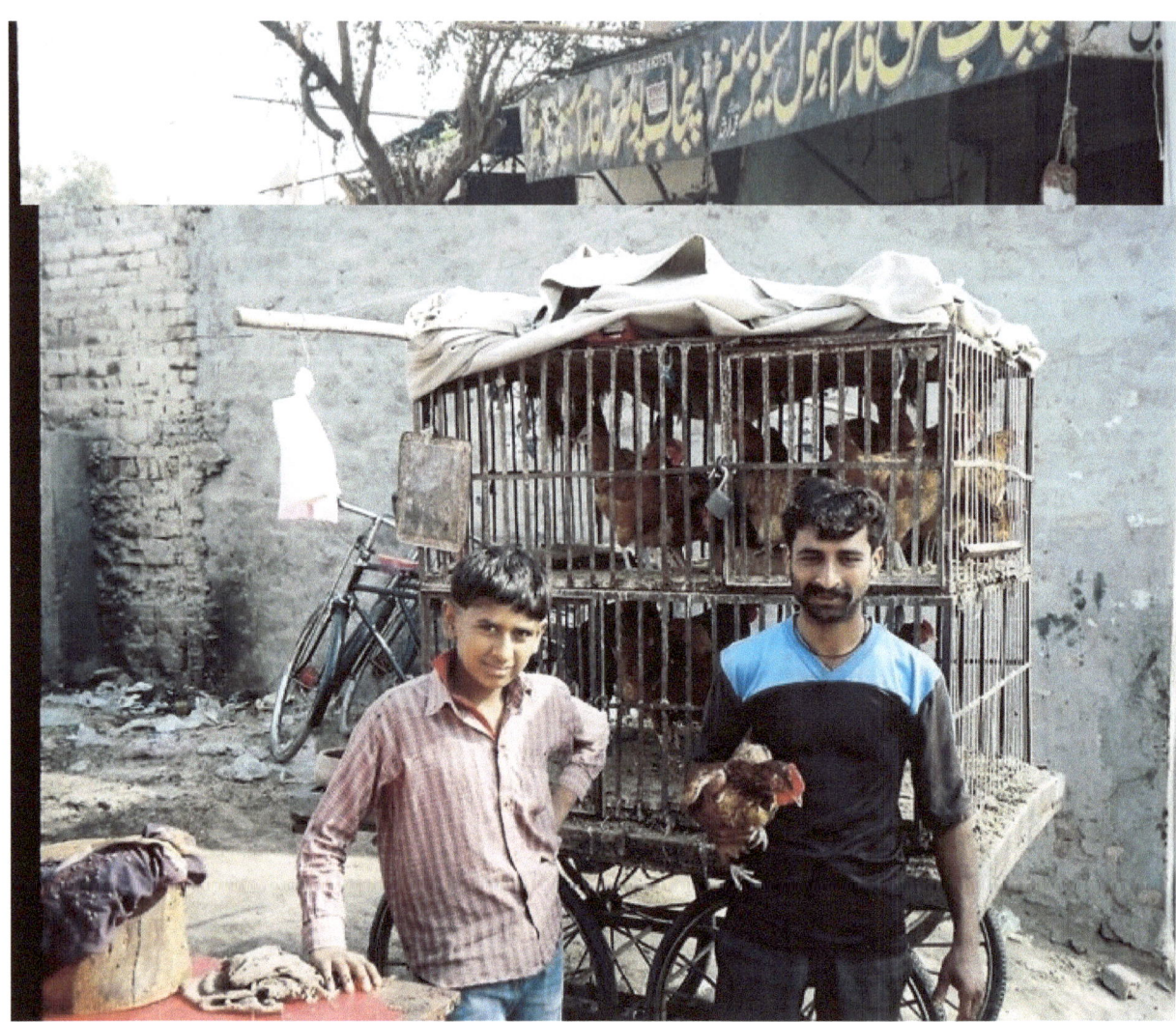

Location

Most of the phatas you will find near or over gutter holes which are open completely or partially with the phata providing the cover standard. They are also found near city disposal sites. City dumps and garbage disposal areas are not good for business so no business will start there the only safe and useful place for a slaughtering poultry phata with less input and more output.

Cleanliness & Hygiene

Cleaniliness in terms of clothes or an apron is not in vogue and not to mention the utensils very old, rotten and usually not very clean. A bucket of water to disperse bacteria and viruses from one carcass to the other while the knife is dipped into the same water bucket routinely. A dirty cloth used to clean the broiler carcass which is also a good transmitting agent of infection. This leads to a complete disrespect for hygiene standards.

Cages

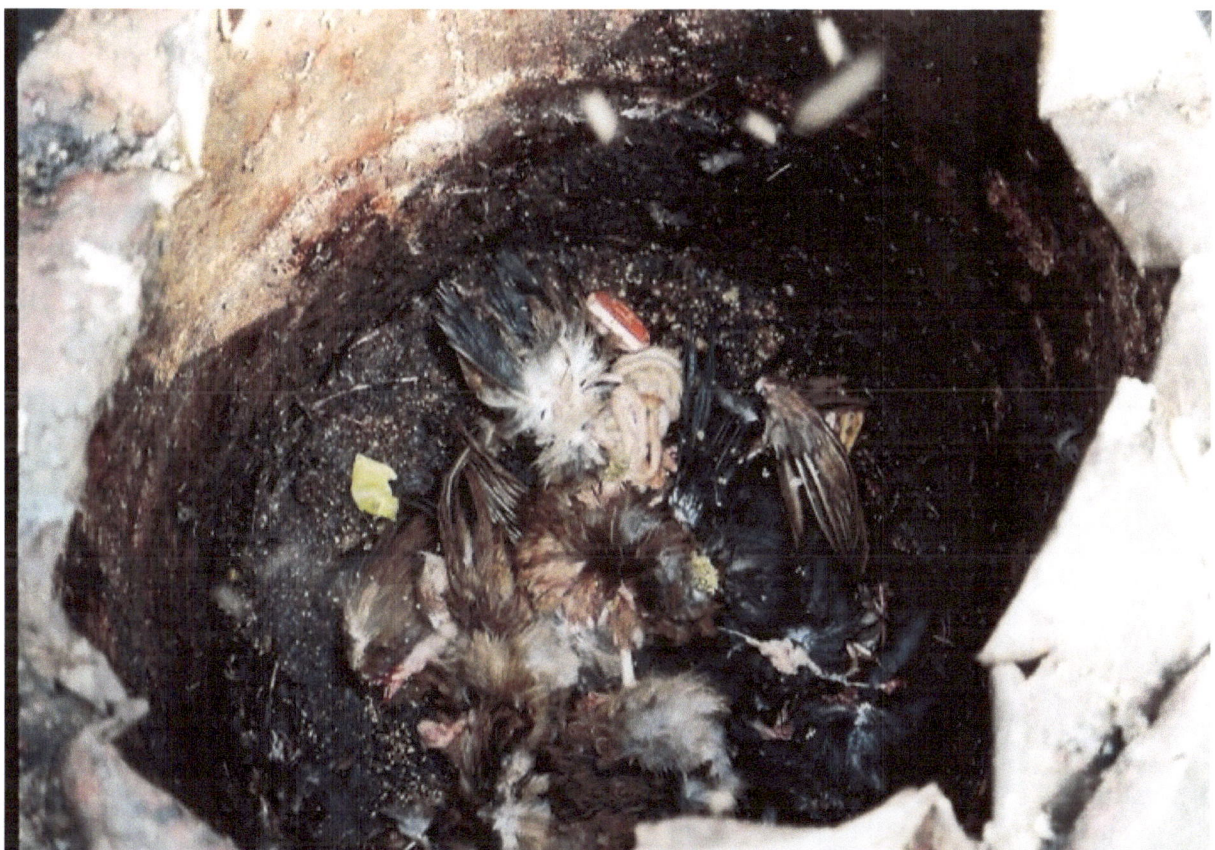

Dirty, rotten, and rusted out cages to hold the live birds and no washing or cleaning technique is used to prevent any dissemination of viruses. That holds true for even the vehicles used to transfer the birds. With no disinfection agent used while their cleaning.

Slaughtering Table

The slaughtering table usually is covered by a plastic sheet which is cleaned by a wet cloth. No disinfection or soaping is not an option to be practices.

Slaughtering tools

Where to begin and where to end I have no clue where the standards start and where they end, better not open this pandora's box.

Slaughtering Temperatures

Complete disregard for the slaughtering temperatures and carcass holding temperatures be it hot and humid weather or the scorching sun of cholistan or the cold inclement weather in December and January. When the rigor mortis starts and when it ends this is usually in the plastic carrier's bag.

Frequent Guests.

Dogs, Cats and mice are the most frequesnt guest at the poultry phata and usually the broiler spare part eating cats and dogs are very docile like the broiler but you never know the hygienic impact of these frequent guests.

Frequent Flyer's

At large and free flight is accorded to the frequent flyer's program which ecompasses, crows, flies and sometimes a sight-seeing swooping kite would make the day more pleasureable.

A request is posted to the higher authorities and the PVMC to make some baseline laws which can control these business entrepreneurships.

REASONS OF MEDICATION AND VACCINATION FAILURES IN PAKISTAN

ONE WORLD-ONE HEALTH

Complete disrespect for this term is being practiced in Pakistan. Physicians and vetrinarians are as apart as anything on solar system from mercury to pluto.

Physicians shun to go to villages and are concentrated in the cities, they don't have any idea about the problems the village folk experience when they live with animals. What is the reaction of villagers they get immune. With nothing to eat and drink and the harsh climate of the weather they become like 'soom' the horses which are trained for battle. There bodies become harsh and stoney and they survive, well survival of the fittest, the unfit move to cities. In the cities the hospitals are jam packed atleast all government hospitals where one infection is transmitted to the other. Even the maulana who speaks and the peer sahib who runs a hepatitis freeing camp in village when it comes to his life he runs to the Doctor's hospital in Lahore. Doctors have started a business entrepreneurship when they did their degree they are into real estate and plaza's after earning from the poor. Since 1947 they number of hospitals built by doctors have increased considerably but built by government I can remember a few. This is not governments fault but the fault of doctors because they don't want to make government hospitals they want to earn in their clinics. The veterinarians role is even worse beaten up at the FSc level they laud they know better than the doctors but infact have an undying emotion of backwardness and humility. You will find in every village a veterinarian on duty but you will seldom find a doctor on call in villages. The treatment of the animal keepers in the villages is left to compounders and they are called doctors. In the villages the munshi of the distributor of feed for poultry is called in when there is a problem with flock and the VA is the one on bike servicing every villager. Where is the philosophy of the pen no one knows. A dental technician is a dental doctor in villages and I have seen barbers doing the duty of the dentists in some villages. There is a solution to this problem.

NO.

ONE HERD-ONE HEALTH

Debate for the next upcoming conference where the scientists will be sleeping. In this telecommunication era Pakistan stands first in the abuse of telecommunication. Prescription via telecom. You have a problem call a doctor tell him what the animal or human is doing and get a prescription via message. What a joke. The writer has experienced it many times that people even educated people call a doctor and take his advice on the telephone. Then the patient expires and we are off to a better doctor who can give advice on telephone. Zareena is sick give zareena's medicine to cow and the cow's medicine to zareena. No one has ever thought of branding or tatoeing or even registering their farmers. No animal is different from the other. No one can tell who has been vaccinated and which has not been counted or vaccinated. No national herd database. Where is the animal who it belongs to or from where it contracted this disease.

The solution to this problem is cull all animal holding of the poor old blind lady with 3 grandchildren 2 goats for milk and 6 bacjyard poultry. We don't know.

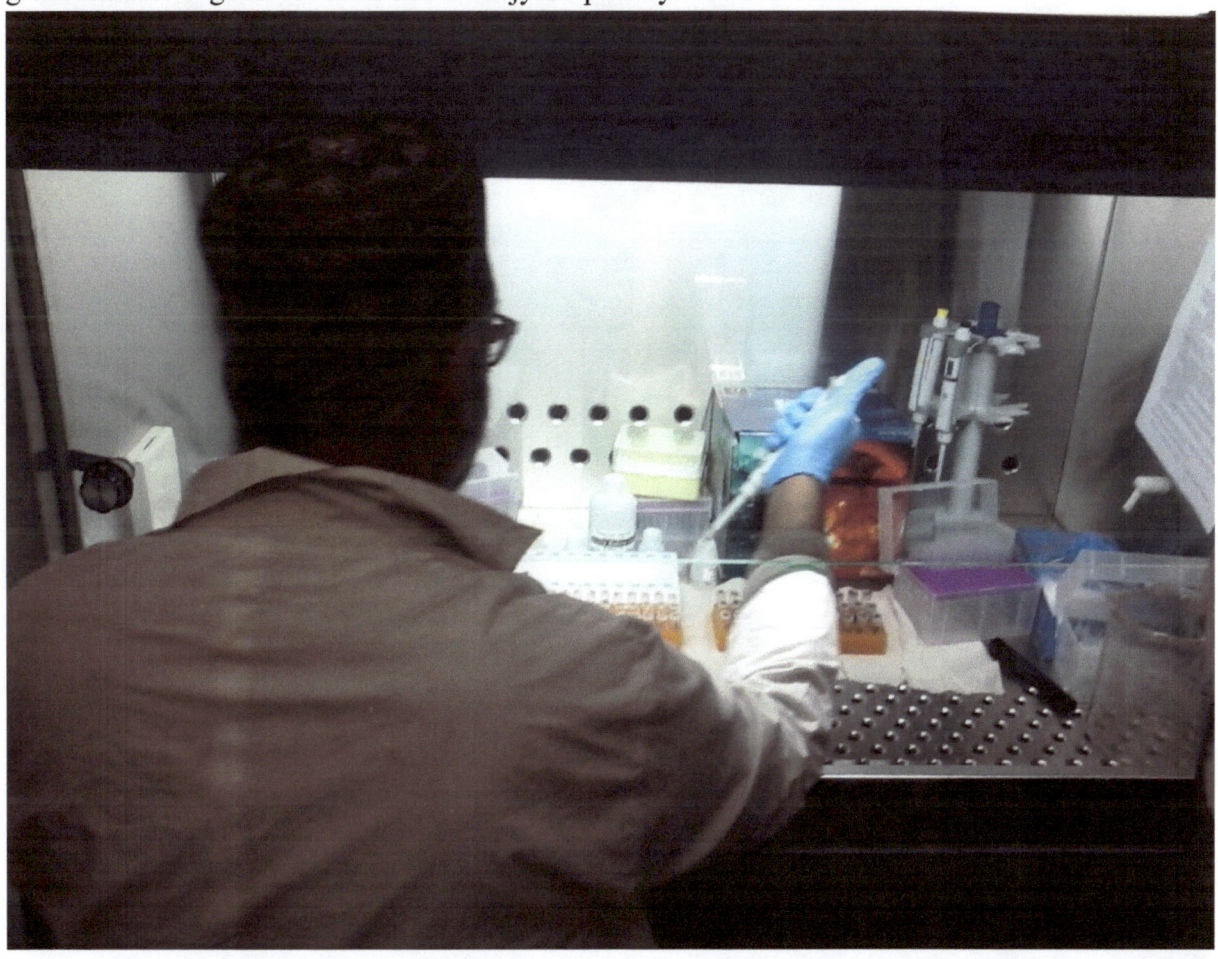

NATIONAL DISEASE DATABASE

At this moment for human and for veterinarians no record is being kept for vaccination, medication and disease. For animals it's a long shot. We don't know when disease outbreaks occur, where they occur and who was affected its all in the hear say, those who stay close and eaves drop get the info correct but mostly incorrect. Otherwise we don't have any database for any person or animal which was healthy or diseased. If we had a national disease databse then the problem would arise of making it available nationwide. Our doctors and veterinarians both have developed a habit of prescribing high potency agents for diseased and resulting in resistance problems.

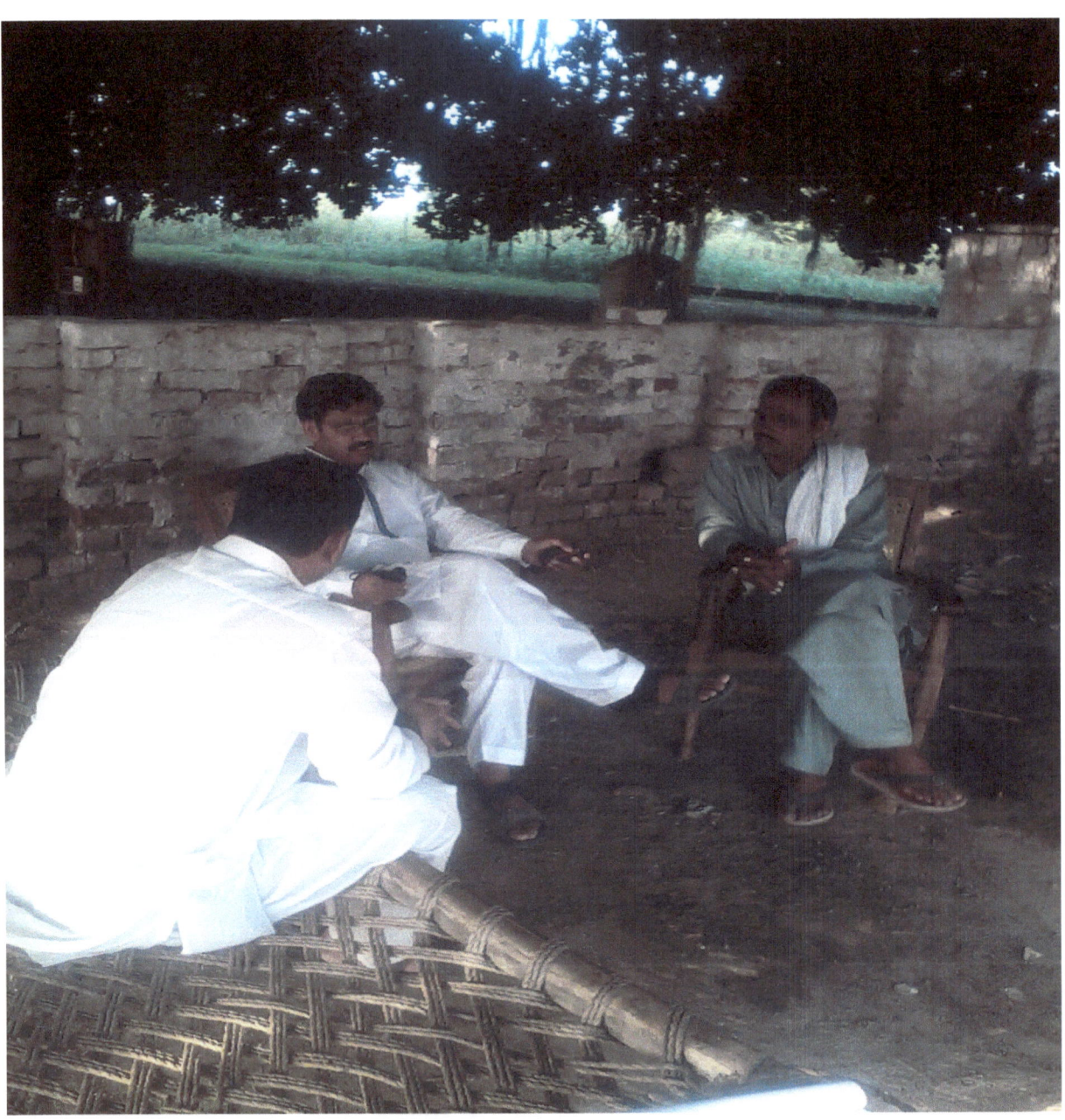

MASS VACCINATION

Mass vaccination is a good thing indeed and is appreciable but when to give first dose and when to administer boosters we have no record for that. We keep on vaccination too pacey then the antibody level decreases to null as is being observed in the case of polio vaccination in humans. Mass vaccination is successful if the whole population is vaccinated but even if foci are left then the vaccines would not work or give false set back figures. Mass vaccination of which population sometimes the host or the reservoirs also need to be vaccinated to control the outbreaks otherwise the reservoirs will lead to sprouting of infections all over the region. Mass vaccination is more fruitful and long lasting in viral infection as far as eradication is concerned the bacterial infections can be controlled but can not be eradicated completely.

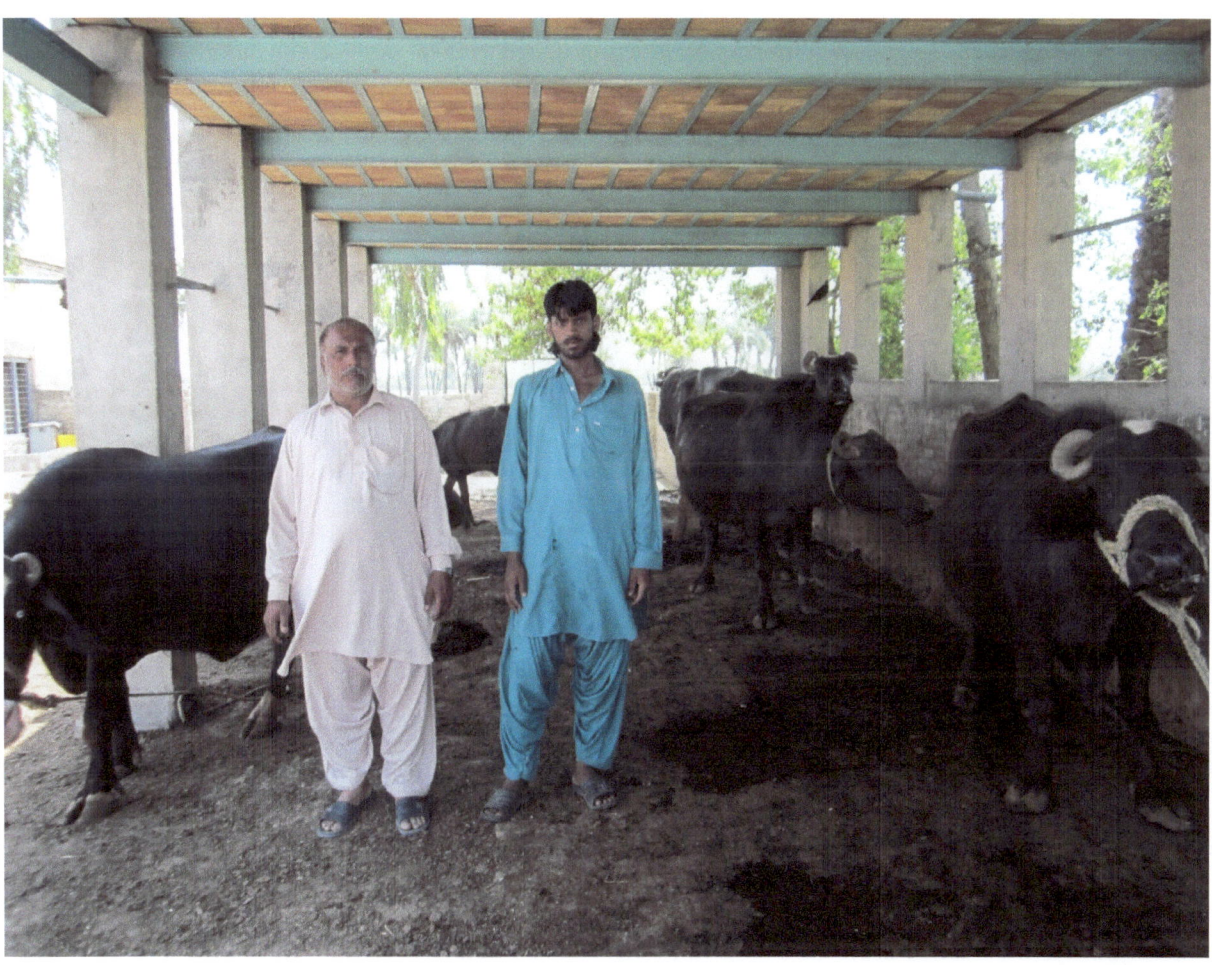

LAB DIAGNOSIS

No one relies on lab diagnosis only few laboratories cater for the whole country. If the laboratories are there they monitor biochemical and physiological parameters for human and nobody has ever gone for disease diagnosis via laboratory. Antibody titers of the herd and animals and humans have never been done oooops sorry we don't have herds sorry.

In poultry sector there is some use of detecting antibody titers and that also is very minimal.

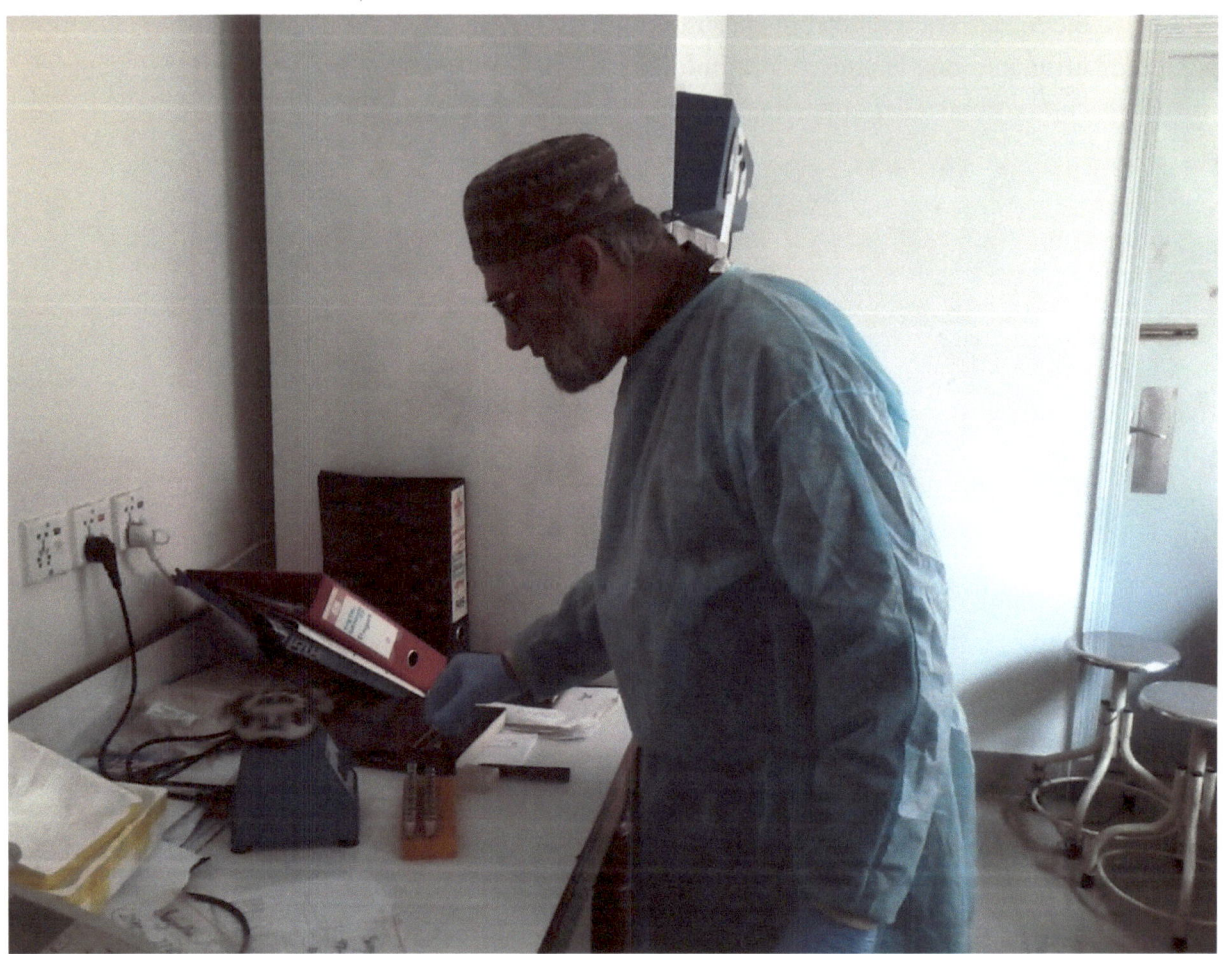

COLD CHANNEL-COLD CHAIN

I don't want to say anything, so many problems with this that I can not waste my time in rephrasing them

MOBILE VETRINARIANS

Mobiles are used by DLO and DDLO for family work and the actual treatment is being done by VA on bike without cold chain for medicines and nor for vaccines.

ELECTRICITY-POWER OUTAGES

There is no electricity in most of the dispensaries be them for human or animal let alone a refrigerator or fridge for cold chain

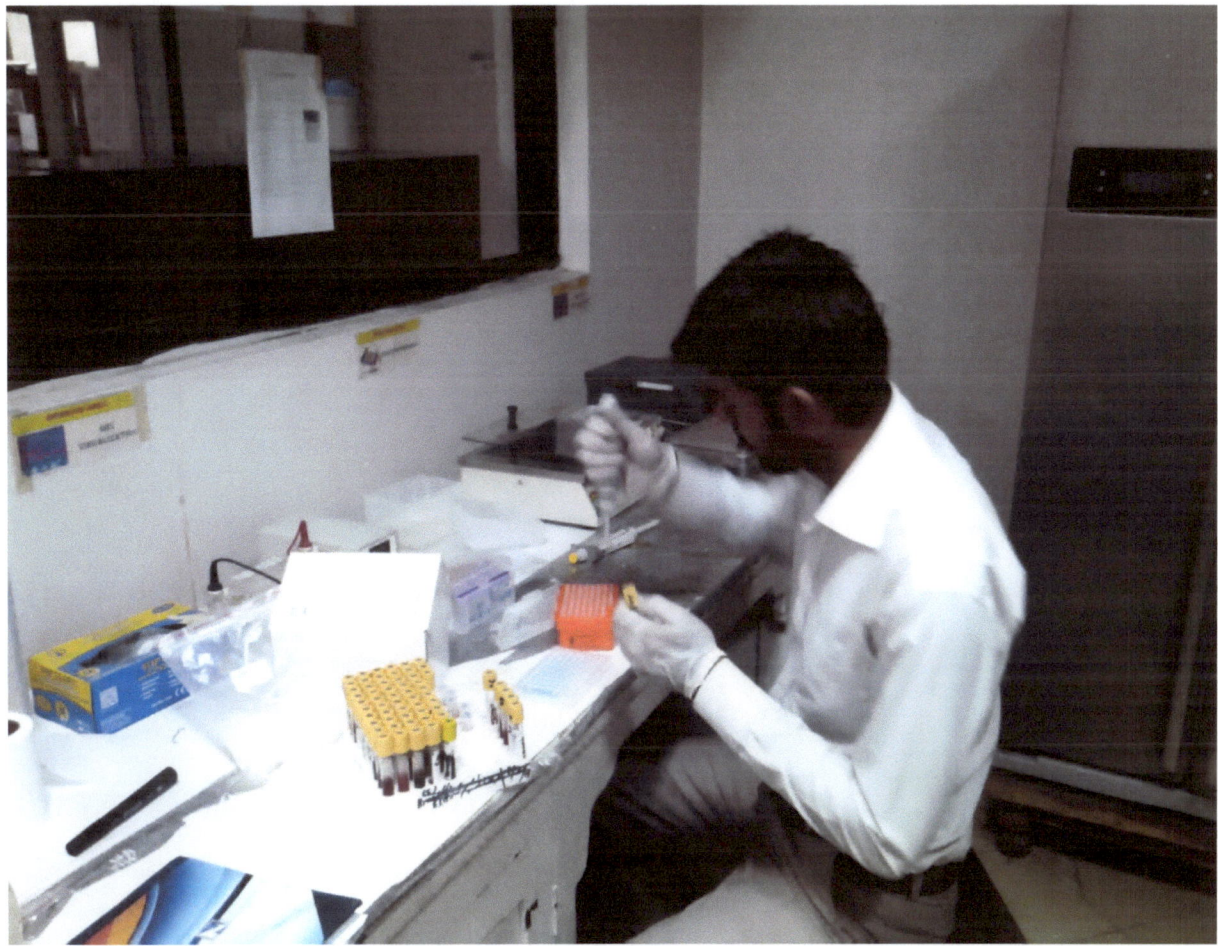

PROFESSIONALLY DISHONEST

Because we want to make money using animal medicines for human health is big business. Because the old lady with three grandchildren and only three goats can not pay so give her an injection mixed with tap water.

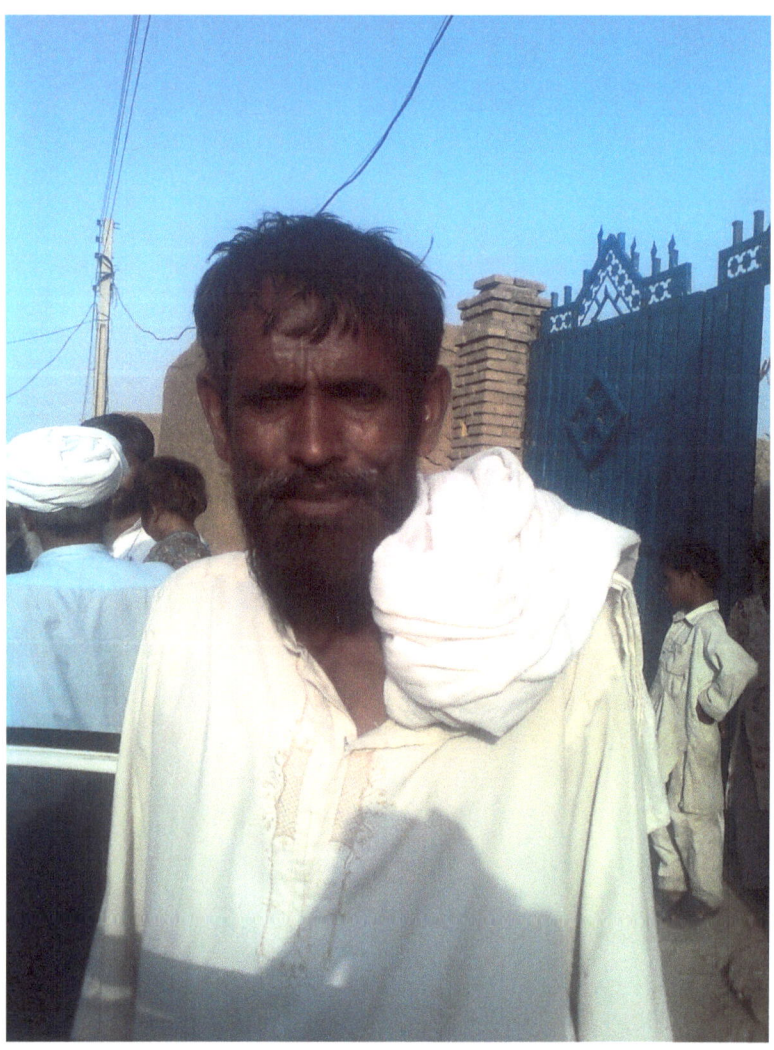

NUTRITION & WATER

The nutrition cake meals storage problems lead to fungal growth and mycotoxins in feed and watering trough are not washed properly leading to algal growths both leading to intoxication.

MASS PRODUCTION

Because we want to do mass vaccination we need more vaccine so quality is compromised because we don't have enough facilities to make vaccines and medicines

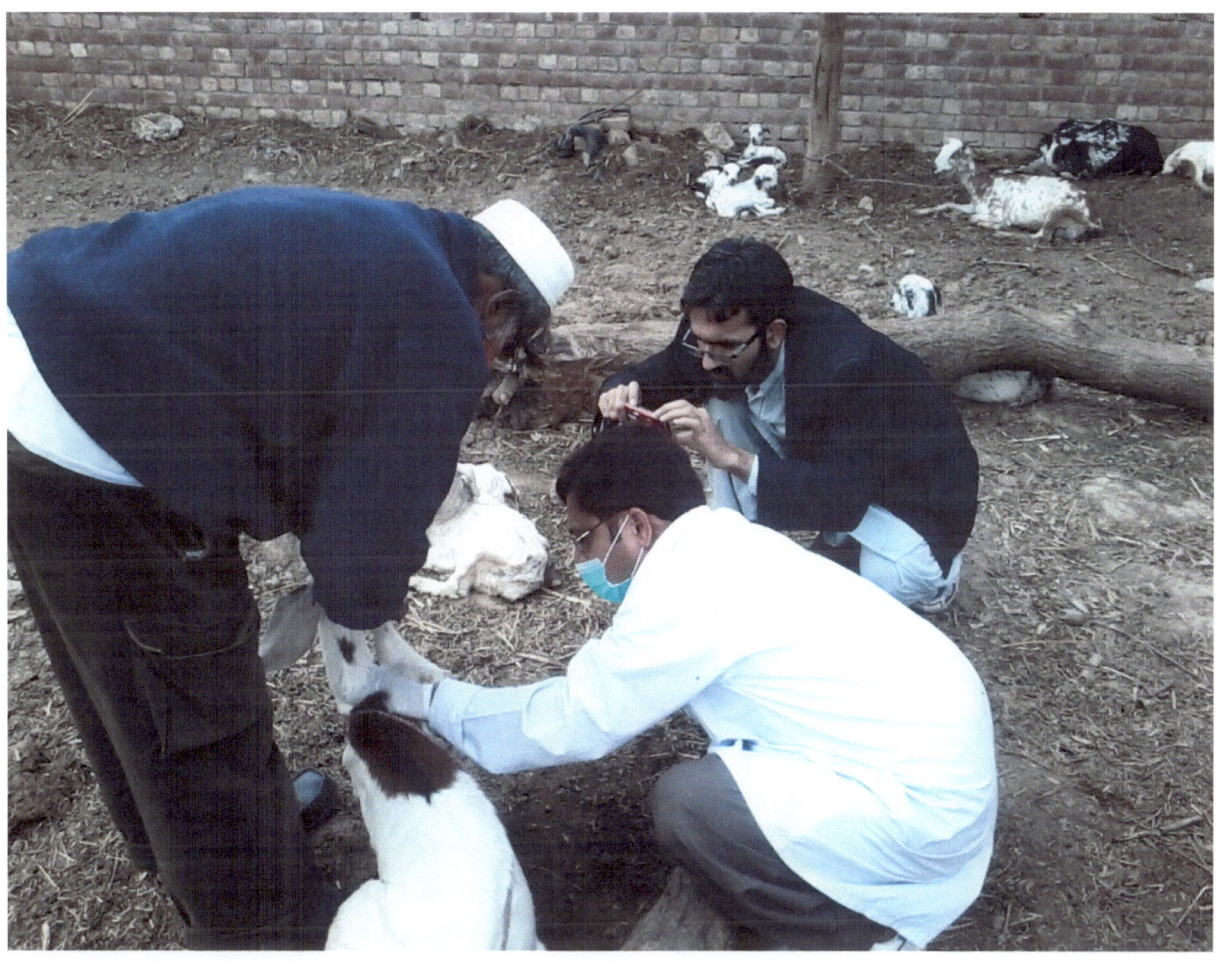

IMPORTATION OF DISEASE

Exotic import leads to import of new germs in them which were not prevalent before.